Table of Contents

How the Body Type Diet Works and How to Know if You're an Endomorph

Endomorphs are primarily characterized by their propensity to store fat, as well as a wider waistline and bigger bone structure, according to the book Integrative Approaches for Health. Endomorphs tend to gain weight more easily compared with ectomorphs and mesomorphs. Even when eating a similar diet as another body type, an endomorph will tend to hold on to more excess fat.

In addition, this excess fat often deposits around the waist. "This visceral body fat hangs out around your organs and is related to insulin resistance," says Marta Montenegro, a certified strength and conditioning specialist (CSCS) and specialist in fitness nutrition in Miami. Insulin resistance is when your cells have trouble responding to the insulin that your pancreas pumps out, which ultimately affects your blood glucose levels, according to the National Institute of Diabetes and Digestive and Kidney Diseases. As Harvard Health Publishing notes,insulin resistance affects the way your body processes carbohydrates. Accordingly, proponents of the endomorph diet advise limiting these, especially highly processed, refined carbs, which contain little or no nutrition, says Montenegro. With more body fat, the thinking goes, you'll also burn fewer calories compared with a naturally muscular body, like a mesomorph.

All this means that you'll have to keep a tighter watch on calories, the diet says. Catudal suggests a higher protein intake (40 percent of calories per day), a good amount of fat (40 percent of calories per day), and a lower-carbohydrate diet (20 percent of calories per day), aiming for 1,300 to 1,500 calories per day to start. Maximize carbs and calories, and build volume by focusing on eating a lot of fiber-rich veggies. "These are the carbs that will keep you full".

Advantages of the Endomorph Diet

Not only do proponents of the endomorph diet say it may help people with this body type lose weight they say it may help their health in other profound ways. Indeed, it's the potential health problems that pose the biggest challenge for endomorphs, says

Melina Jampolis, MD, an internist and board-certified physician nutrition specialist in Valley Village, California. "An endomorph likely has a genetic component to being a bit heavier. If you look at somatotypes, many people with [type 2] diabetes are considered to be endomorphs," she says.

But even if you're considered overweight, it's more important to look at where you're carrying this fat. If excess fat lands on your hips, thighs, and butt (a classic pear shape), you likely have fewer risk factors for metabolic disease compared with someone who stores fat in their midsection (a classic apple). Metabolic syndrome is a cluster of risk factors a large waistline, inactivity, insulin resistance that raise your risk for heart disease and stroke, according to the National Heart, Lung, and Blood Institute. (9) Insulin resistance is often present in those who have prediabetes and type 2 diabetes, raising blood glucose levels slightly (but not high enough to be full-blown diabetes). "When you carry weight in your belly, you're more than likely less responsive to insulin compared to someone who carries weight more diffusely through their body," says Dr. Jampolis.

In fact, in a June 2015 study in PLOS Medicine, researchers concluded that waist circumference was predictive of type 2 diabetes in overweight and obese adults. The link was even stronger in women. Following a body type diet for an endomorph may help you adopt healthy eating patterns and exercise to improve insulin sensitivity and lose fat (particularly visceral fat) that may be putting your health at risk. That said, Jampolis doesn't agree with dieting for your somatotype. But when you move toward a healthier pattern of eating and for someone with excess fat around their waist it could be reducing overall carb intake you can trim your waistline to reduce your risk for health problems. Focus on your waist circumference (rather than hitting a specific goal weight): Women should have a waist that's under 35 inches; for men, that's 40 inches, according to the Centers for Disease Control and Prevention

Disadvantages of the Endomorph Diet

Besides there being a lack of large, long-term studies on the endomorph diet and the body type diet as a whole, this eating plan can pose some challenges that may prove insurmountable for some people.

First comes the hurdle of cutting carbs.

Because of a potential overproduction of insulin, your body likely doesn't manage carbs as well as the other body types. "I tell patients to eat lower levels of carbs and more healthy fats, particularly monounsaturated fatty acids," says Jampolis. Examples of monounsaturated fats (MUFAs) are nuts, avocado, and olive oil, according to Medline Plus. "It's also especially important to make most or all grains whole grain," she says.

The problem arises because while it's easy to tell someone to eat less bread, rice, pasta, crackers, and potatoes, it can be more difficult to put the rule into practice, especially if you're accustomed to eating this way. That may make this type of diet more difficult to stick to for some folks. For instance, while a past study found that people with type 2 diabetes who followed a low-carb diet lost weight and were able to lower their insulin medication, they also discovered that they were unlikely to stick to the diet after six months.

Foods to eat and avoid

Sources differ on what the best endomorph diet plan is.

Generally, people with endomorphic bodies may benefit from a nutrition plan that balances healthful fats, proteins, and carbohydrates from fruits, vegetables, and unrefined, high fiber foods.

Some examples of foods that are rich in protein or healthful monounsaturated and polyunsaturated fats include:

- low fat dairy products, such as low fat milk, yogurt, and cheeses
- poultry, such as chicken and turkey
- most types of fish, especially fatty fish
- most nontropical vegetable cooking oils, especially olive, canola, and avocado oil
- eggs and egg whites
- most nontropical nuts, including almonds, hazelnuts, and walnuts

Some examples of carbohydrates that are fit for an endomorph diet include most:

- dried beans and legumes, such as kidney beans, lentils, and chickpeas
- fruits, except melons and pineapple
- non-starchy vegetables, such as broccoli, cauliflower, and celery
- whole-grain or whole-wheat products, such as all-bran cereal and 100% stone-ground whole-wheat bread
- some starchy vegetables, such as sweet potatoes, yams, corn, and carrots
- some unrefined starchy vegetables, such as quinoa and amaranth

According to the American Council on Exercise (ACE), people with an endomorph body type tend to be more sensitive to carbohydrates and insulin. Insulin is a hormone that allows blood sugars to enter cells.

So, people following an endomorph diet may wish to limit or avoid carbohydrate dense foods, especially refined carbohydrates such as white flour and sugar.

Foods rich in carbohydrates release sugars rapidly into the bloodstream, causing blood sugar spikes and dips. The body is also more likely to turn these sugars into fat than burn them as energy.

Endomorphic bodies are also more likely to convert excess calories into fat. For this same reason, people following an endomorph diet may also want to avoid foods that are calorie dense but nutrient poor.

Some examples of foods to limit or avoid on the endomorph diet include:

- white bread, white rice, traditional pasta, and bagels
- candies, chocolates, and other sweets
- baked goods and cakes
- soft drinks, energy drinks, and sports drinks
- refined cereals, such as bran flakes, instant oatmeal, and puffed rice
- heavily processed or fried foods
- rich dairy products, such as cream, whipped cream, and ice cream
- red meats
- foods rich in sodium
- alcohol
- cooking oils with a lot of saturated fat, such as palm or coconut oil

A 7-Day Sample Menu for the Endomorph Body Type

DAY 1

Breakfast 2 scrambled eggs plus 1 egg white and spinach

Snack Sunflower seeds and a piece of fruit

Lunch Olive oil–massaged kale salad topped with cucumbers, bell peppers, and salmon

Snack Deli meat wrapped around asparagus spears

Dinner Grilled chicken breast over zucchini noodles and tomato sauce

DAY 2

Breakfast Cottage cheese with slivered almonds and cinnamon

Snack Sliced veggies and hummus

Lunch Stir-fry made with chicken and peppers over brown rice

Snack Sliced apple with peanut butter

Dinner Turkey tacos wrapped in lettuce and topped with a slice of avocado

DAY 3

Breakfast Egg frittata made with tomatoes, onions, and spinach

Snack Protein shake

Lunch Grilled chicken salad with garbanzo beans, tomatoes, and tzatziki sauce

Snack Hummus and sliced veggies (bell pepper, celery)

Dinner White fish drizzled in olive oil, roasted broccoli and cauliflower

DAY 4

Breakfast Smoothie made with Greek yogurt, berries, and almond milk

Snack Sliced veggies and hummus

Lunch Open-faced turkey, veggie, and avocado sandwich on whole-wheat toast

Snack Pistachios and cubed cantaloupe

Dinner Sliced steak stir-fry over cauliflower rice

DAY 5

Breakfast Omelet made with peppers and spinach, topped with avocado slices

Snack Protein bar

Lunch Quinoa mixed with chopped veggies and cubed chicken breast, tossed with vinaigrette

Snack Carrots dipped in peanut butter

Dinner Salmon, steamed broccoli, sautéed mushrooms

DAY 6

Breakfast 2 hard-boiled eggs with blueberries

Snack Greek yogurt with sliced almonds

Lunch Mediterranean lentil salad with sun-dried tomatoes, kalamata olives, and chopped raw veggies

Snack Protein shake

Dinner Veggie and bean soup with a grilled chicken breast

DAY 7

Breakfast Greek yogurt layered with apples, cinnamon, and walnuts

Snack Hard-boiled egg and sliced avocado

Lunch Sweet potato stuffed with shredded chicken, drizzled with low-sugar barbecue sauce

Snack Hummus and veggies

Dinner Shrimp and veggie kabobs with cauliflower rice

Endomorph exercises

Exercise is an important part of any weight loss plan, especially for people with an endomorph body type. Exercising helps increase metabolism and reduce fat.

Cardiovascular exercises such as running can burn calories and help create a calorie deficit. This means that someone is using more calories than they are consuming and potentially burning excess fat.

The ACE recommend that people with an endomorph body type follow "well rounded" exercise routines that focus on both cardiovascular and strength training activities.

Some examples of good cardiovascular exercises include:

- High intensity interval training (HIIT): In HIIT, a person will alternate between periods of very high intensity exercise and low intensity exercise or rest. Those with endomorphic bodies can try doing HIIT sessions two or three times per week for a maximum of 30 minutes per session.
- Steady state training (SST): These are longer sessions of consistent moderate to low intensity exercise. Good SST exercises include walking, jogging, and swimming. People with an endomorph body type can try doing 30–60-minute SST sessions two to three times per week.

Building muscle

Deadlift is a good example of a compound exercise to build muscle.

Strength and weight training exercises are an important part of almost any weight loss plan, especially for people with an endomorph body type. These people often have a low percentage of muscle mass, although they have large, wide bones typically capable of bearing large, strong muscles. They also tend to have excess body fat, which triggers the body to release estrogen, reducing testosterone levels and hindering muscle growth. However, healthy muscle helps increase metabolism, because unlike fat cells, muscle tissues burn calories, even when resting. They also encourage the body to use fat for fuel.

Several weight training routines and exercises are beneficial for people with endomorphic bodies. For example, experts tend to recommend compound exercises. Compound exercises use multiple body tissues and units at the same time and encourage body control. People can do most of these exercises from a standing position using free weights, body weight, or a barbell.

Some examples of compound exercises include:

Deadlift or hip hinge

To do:

1. Stand with the legs hip-width apart and close to the barbell.

2. Drive the hips back while bracing the core, keeping tension in the back and the knees soft, and pushing the heels into the floor.

3. As the bar reaches the knees, try shooting the hips into the bar.

5. Finish standing tall while clenching the glutes.

Pushups

To do:

1. Place the hands on the floor, with the fingers spread widely, directly below the shoulders.

2. Pack the shoulders while squeezing the glutes and pressing the heels away.

3. Keeping the head in line with the body, bend the elbows, and lower the chest toward the floor with control.

5. Keep the back straight then engage the legs, glutes, and shoulders to raise the chest back up.

Squats

To do:

1. Standing with the legs shoulder-width apart, drive the feet into the floor and activate the hips.

2. Slowly, and with control, lower the tailbone toward the floor with a tall and engaged torso.

4. Once lowered, slowly push the body away from the floor until standing tall with the torso fully extended.

Circuit training

Another group of strength exercises that experts recommend for people with an endomorph body type is circuit training.

Circuit training involves doing short, intense bouts of exercise with small periods of rest in-between.

One example of circuit training may involve:

1. squat with overhead press (50 seconds)

2. rest (10 seconds)

3. stationary lunge with lateral raise, right leg front (50 seconds)

4. rest (10 seconds)

5. stationary lunge with lateral raise, left leg front holding dumbbells (50 seconds)

6. rest (10 seconds)

7. plié squat or upright row, dumbbells or kettlebell (50 seconds)

8. rest (10 seconds)

9. pushups with single leg knee drives (50 seconds)

10. rest (10 seconds)

11. plank with triceps extension, dumbbells (50 seconds)

12. rest (10 seconds)

13. alternate step-ups with hammer curls, dumbbells (50 seconds)

14. repeat these steps three times

Healthy Soba Noodles Recipes

Ingredients

- 1 pack soba noodles
- Water for boiling
- Salt to taste

Preparation

- Bring a large pot of water to boil on the stove.
- Add salt to the water before adding the soba noodles.

- Cook until the noodles become soft, but be careful, as the noodles can easily overcook and become mushy.
- Drain the water and run the pasta under cold water immediately (if you want the noodles for a cold dish).

GARDEN VEGGIE FRITTATA

Ingredients

- 1 teaspoon olive oil
- cooking spray
- ¾ cup broccoli florets cut into 1-inch pieces
- 1 red bell pepper cut into ½ inch pieces
- ¼ cup chopped red onion

- 4 eggs
- 4 egg whites
- 1/3 cup shredded or diced cheddar cheese or cheese variety of your choice
- fresh herbs for garnish such as chopped cilantro parsley or green onion
- salt and pepper to taste

Preparation

- Preheat the oven to 400 degrees. Heat the oil in an 8-inch pan over medium-high heat.
- Add the red onion to the pan and cook, stirring occasionally, for 3-4 minutes or until onion has softened.

- Add the red pepper and cook for another 3 minutes or until the pepper has softened.
- Add the broccoli to the pan along with 1 tablespoon of water and cook, stirring occasionally, until broccoli is tender.
- Season the vegetables to taste with salt and pepper.
- Remove the vegetables from the pan and wipe the pan clean with a paper towel.
- Coat the pan with cooking spray.
- In a bowl whisk together the eggs and egg whites, season to taste with salt and pepper.
- Add the vegetables and cheese to the egg mixture and stir until combined.
- Pour the egg mixture into the pan and place in the oven.

- Bake for 15 minutes or until center is set. Garnish with fresh herbs, cut into wedges and serve.

Instant Pot Weight Loss Soup

Ingredients

- 1 tablespoon extra-virgin olive oil
- 2 medium onions (chopped)
- 4 medium carrots (chopped)
- 4 stalks celery (chopped)
- 4 cloves garlic (minced)
- 4 cups chopped cabbage (half head)
- 1 green bell pepper (chopped)
- 1 zucchini (chopped)
- 1 14- ounce can diced tomatoes

- 8 cups bone broth (or low-sodium vegetable broth)
- 1 bay leaf
- 1 teaspoon oregano
- 1 teaspoon basil
- ½ teaspoon red pepper flakes
- 1 teaspoon salt (optional)
- 1/2 teaspoon black pepper

Preparation

- Set Instant Pot to the saute setting. Add the olive oil and allow to heat for 1 minute. Add the onion, carrots and celery and cook, stirring occasionally, until softened, 5 -7 minutes. Stir in the garlic and cook for 1 minute longer.

- Add the cabbage, green pepper, zucchini, tomatoes, broth, bay leaf, spices and salt and pepper. Stir to combine.
- Put the lid on the Instant Pot, close the steam vent and set to HIGH pressure using the manual setting. Decrease the time to 4 minutes. It will take about 15 minutes for the pressure to build, then the timer will start.
- Once the time is expired, wait for 5 minutes, then carefully use the quick release valve to release the steam. Season to taste with salt and pepper. Serve.

For the stovetop:

- Heat the olive oil in a large saucepan set over medium heat. Add the onion, carrots and celery and cook, stirring occasionally, until softened, about 5 minutes. Stir in the garlic and cook for 1 minute longer.
- Add the cabbage, green pepper, zucchini, tomatoes, broth, bay leaf, spices and salt and pepper. Stir to combine.
- Bring to a boil, then reduce heat and simmer for 20 minutes, stirring occasionally.
- Season to taste with salt and pepper. Serve.

Jump-Start Your Day Breakfast Burritos

Ingredients

- 2 teaspoons olive oil
- 1 small yellow onion, chopped
- 1 red bell pepper, chopped
- Kosher salt and black pepper
- 1 cup canned black beans, drained and rinsed
- 1 teaspoon chili powder
- 6 whole eggs plus 6 egg whites
- ½ cup shredded reduced fat cheddar cheese
- 6 (9-inch) whole grain wraps (I used La Tortilla Factory Smart Delicious Whole Grain Soft Wraps)
- ¾ cup your favorite salsa

- ¼ cup sliced scallions
- Hot sauce (optional)

Preparation

- Heat the oil in a large nonstick skillet over medium heat. Add the onions and peppers to the skillet and season them with salt and pepper. Cook, stirring occasionally, until softened, 7-8 minutes. Stir in the beans and chili powder and cook another 2-3 minutes until heated through. Pour the contents of the skillet into a bowl and set aside. Wipe the skillet clean.
- Whisk the eggs and egg whites together in a large bowl along with ½ teaspoon salt and ¼ teaspoon black pepper. Spray the skillet with nonstick

cooking spray and heat over medium heat. Add the eggs and cook them, stirring occasionally, until soft curds form. Stir in the cheese and cook another minute until melted. Remove from heat.

- Spread each tortilla with equal amounts of the veggie/bean mixture and top with the scrambled eggs. Spread 2 tablespoons salsa, some sliced scallions and hot sauce (if using) on top. Roll the tortillas up burrito style- fold the side closest to you over the filling, then fold both sides in toward the center and roll up. Serve alone or with reduced fat sour cream, if desired.
- If not eating right away, wrap each burrito in plastic wrap or aluminum foil and freeze. To reheat, unwrap and

microwave until warm, about 2 minutes, turning over halfway through. For a crispier wrapping, heat in the microwave, then bake in a 450° oven for 5 to 10 minutes.

Lemony Roasted Low-Carb Broccoli

Ingredients

- 2 cups chopped broccoli
- 1 tablespoon olive oil
- 1/2 teaspoon sea salt
- 1 large lemon, peeled and juiced
- 1/4 teaspoon crushed red pepper flakes

- 1/8 teaspoon oregano

Preparation

- Preheat oven to 375F. Line a baking sheet with tin foil. In a large mixing bowl, combine broccoli florets with oil, salt, lemon juice, lemon peel, red pepper flakes, and oregano. Mix all the ingredients together until thoroughly combined. Pour the broccoli mixture onto the lined baking sheet and spread out in one even layer. Bake at 375F for 20 minutes or until broccoli is lightly browned and crispy, flipping the mixture once halfway through. Remove from oven and enjoy hot or at room temperature.

SWEET POTATO AND CHICKEN HASH

INGREDIENTS

- 1 tbsp ghee
- 2 boneless skinless chicken breasts, (about 300g each)
- 1 medium sweet potato, peeled and spiralized (about 350g)
- 1 gala apple, cored and diced
- 1 cup water, divided
- 1 cup baby spinach leaves, chopped
- 2 tbsp organic raisins
- 1/2 tsp Himalayan salt
- 1/2 tsp ground black pepper
- 1 tsp garam masala
- 1/4 tsp freshly ground nutmeg

Preparation

- Melt the ghee in a large skillet placed over medium-high heat. Once the fat is nice and hot, add the chicken and cook until golden brown, about 6 to 8 minutes total.
- Add 1/2 cup water and deglaze the pan, then stir in salt, pepper, garam masala and freshly ground nutmeg.
- Add the apple and sauté for about one minute, or until the apple is slightly softened.
- Throw in the spiralized sweet potato, add another 1/2 cup of water and cook, stirring delicately until the sweet potato is soft and water is almost completely evaporated.

- Kill the heat, throw in the chopped spinach and raisins. Stir delicately until the ingredients are evenly distributed and spinach is sufficiently wilted.
- Serve without delay.

Green Monster Smoothie

INGREDIENTS

- 1 cup plain or vanilla coconut milk (I use Silk Brand PureCoconut)
- 6-8 oz vanilla greek yogurt
- 1 RIPE, frozen banana
- 2-4 cups raw, organic spinach (I use 3 cups)

Preparation

- Place all ingredients into a blender.
- Blend & liquify
- Serve

Strawberry Spinach Salad

INGREDIENTS

- 4 cups baby spinach
- 1 cup strawberries sliced lengthwise
- ¼ cup chopped walnuts
- 1 cup precooked rotisserie chicken shredded –optional-
- 3 tablespoons crumbled cheese such as Chevre feta or blue cheese

- Strawberry citrus vinaigrette
- 5 strawberries quartered
- ¼ cup orange juice
- 1/4 cup white wine vinegar or apple cider vinegar
- 3 tablespoons extra virgin olive oil

Preparation

- Make the vinaigrette ahead of time, combine all the ingredients in a blender and blend until smooth. Move to a jar and place in the fridge for 1-4 hours to marinate.
- Cover a large platter with baby spinach, then top with strawberries, walnuts and chicken.

- Drizzle half the dressing over the spinach, place the rest of the dressing next to the salad.
- Top with cheese, freshly grated pepper and serve with Opolo pinot gris
- NOTE- If you choose to take this Strawberry Spinach Salad salad with you on a picnic or potluck, place the spinach in a large Tupperware container, cover with 2 layers of paper towels and close.
- Add the chicken, strawberries, walnuts and cheese to small containers or bags and leave the vinaigrette in the jar to take along, now you're ready for a fabulous picnic or potluck. Just open the spinach container and top with all the fixings and you're set in a matter of seconds.

Rice Cakes with Peanut Butter

Ingredients

- 1 ½ tablespoons peanut butter
- 2 multigrain rice cakes

Preparation

- Step 1 Divide peanut butter between rice cakes and spread evenly.

Salmon Burgers with Jicama Mango Slaw

Ingredients

- For Salmon Burgers:
- 16 oz salmon filets, skin removed
- 2 eggs
- 3/4 cup almond meal
- 1/3 cup red onion, minced
- 3 garlic cloves, minced
- 1/2 cup cilantro, finely chopped
- Sea salt and black pepper, to taste
- 2 T olive oil for cooking
- For Jicama Mango Slaw:
- 2 cups green cabbage, shredded
- 1 cup jicama, julienned
- 1 cup mango, diced
- 1/2 cup red onion, thinly sliced

- 1/4 cup fresh lime juice
- 2 T olive oil
- 1/3 cup cilantro, minced
- Sea salt to taste

Preparation

- Begin by finely chopping the salmon filets and add to a large mixing bowl. Add the rest of the burger ingredients and stir to combine.
- Form mixture into patties. Set onto a plate.
- Heat olive oil in a large pan over medium heat. Allow pan to become very hot. Place salmon burgers on pan. Use spatula to reform patties if

they become loose. Cook 5 minutes. Flip and cook 5 minutes on other side.
- While burgers cook, make the slaw by combining cabbage, red onion, mango, jicama and cilantro in a large bowl. Pour in lime juice and olive oil. Season with sea salt. Toss to coat. Refrigerate until serving.
- Serve salmon patties with slaw.

Spicy Sausage & Cabbage Skillet Melt

Ingredients

- 4 links spicy Italian chicken sausages
- 1 ½ cups green cabbage, shredded
- 1 ½ cups purple cabbage, shredded
- ½ cup onion, diced

- 2 Tbsp. coconut oil
- 2 slices Colby Jack cheese, (1 ounce each)
- 2 Tbsp. cilantro, fresh and chopped

Preparation

- Remove casings from sausages and rough chop. Chop onion and shred cabbage if not using pre-shredded cabbage.
- Melt coconut oil in a large skillet and add onion and cabbage. Cook over medium-high heat until the vegetables begin to become tender, about 8 minutes.

- Add sausage, stirring to mix it into the cabbage and onions. Cook 8 minutes more.
- Add the cheese on top and cover the skillet.
- Turn off the heat and wait 5 minutes while the cheese melts into the cabbage and vegetables.
- Remove the lid from the skillet and stir. Top with cilantro and serve immediately right from the skillet

AVOCADO CHICKEN SALAD

Ingredients

- 2 cups poached chicken finely diced (10 oz)
- 1 medium Hass Avocado, mashed
- 1/3 cup celery, finely diced (1 large rib)
- 2 tbsp red onion or scallion, minced
- 2 tbsp cilantro, finely chopped
- 2 tbsp avocado oil (or your favorite)
- 1 tbsp fresh lemon juice (or lime juice)
- salt and pepper to taste

Preparation

- Prepare the celery, onion, and cilantro, placing in a medium bowl. Dice the chicken and add it to the bowl with the vegetables.

- Cut into the avocado with a chef's knife until the blade hits the pit. Slide the knife around the pit, cutting the avocado in half. Twist the halves to separate. Remove the pit by tapping the knife into the pit until it sticks, make sure the avocado half is held steadily on a cutting board before attempting. Scoop out the avocado flesh with a spoon and place into a small bowl. Mash with a fork until smooth and creamy. Stir in the lemon juice and oil.

- Add the mashed avocado to the to the chicken and vegetables and stir to mix. Serve over lettuce or enjoy on a low carb bagel.
- Makes 3, 3/4-1 cup servings.

LOW CARB SPAGHETTI SQUASH SHRIMP SCAMPI

INGREDIENTS

- 1 squash, spaghetti style
- 1 lb shrimp, shells removed, cleaned, and deveined
- ½ cup butter
- ¼ cup garlic, minced
- ½ cup white whine, dry

- 1 tsp red pepper flakes
- 1 tbsp dried oregano
- 1 tbsp dried thyme
- 1 tbsp dried parsley

Preparation

- Preheat oven to 350 degrees.
- Slice spaghetti squash in half, scoop out stringy pulp and seeds, discard.
- Place halves, face up, on baking sheet.
- Pour water on bottom of baking sheet.
- Place pats of butter in squash halves.
- Bake 40 minutes to an hour, until squash is tender to the touch. If squash is not yet tender, continue to cook.

- When squash is soft, remove from oven and let cool until it is comfortable to handle, about 20 minutes.
- While squash is cooling, start cooking shrimp scampi.
- In a large pan, melt butter and add garlic on medium heat.
- Cook until garlic is fragrant and soft, about 3 minutes.
- When butter is melted, add shrimp, spices, and wine, and cook until shrimp is pink and opaque, about 8 minutes, stirring often.
- While shrimp is cooking, run a fork through squash to form spaghetti-like strings.
- Shred squash all the way to bottom of squash rind - but do not pierce rind (if serving in the rind as a "boat").

- When shrimp is cooked, add squash "spaghetti" strings to pan and toss over high heat until well mixed.
- Spoon back into squash rind "boats".
- Top with parsley and parmesan cheese.
- Serve Immediately.

MALANGA, BLACK BEAN AND PEPPER SALAD

INGREDIENTS

- 1 lb malanga, root peeled, cut into 1/2-inch pieces (about 2 roots)
- 2 cups chicken broth or 2 cups beef broth
- 1 (15 ounce) can black beans, drained

* 1 cup chopped roasted red pepper
* RED ONION CILANTRO VINAIGRETTE
* 1/4 cup olive oil or 1/4 cup vegetable oil
* 1/4 cup lime juice or 1/4 cup lemon juice
* 1/4 cup minced red onion
* 2 tablespoons chopped fresh cilantro
* 2 garlic cloves, minced
* 1/2 teaspoon salt
* 1/4 teaspoon red pepper flakes

Preparation

* Boil the malanga in the broth, partially covered, until tender, about 15 minutes; drain.

- Combine the malanga, black beans
  and roasted peppers in a large bowl.
- Combine dressing ingredients in a jar
  or bowl and mix well. Pour over salad.
  Chill for up to 24 hours.

Keto Cream Cheese Frosting

INGREDIENTS

- 8 ounces cream cheese, softened
- 1/2 cup (1 stick) butter, softened
- 2/3 cup powdered erythritol (I used
  Swerve)
- 1/2 teaspoon vanilla extract (no sugar
  added)

Preparation

- In a medium bowl, cream the butter and cream cheese together with a mixer until fully combined.
- Add the sweetener and vanilla extract and beat slowly until the sweetener is incorporated so it doesn't get blown into the air.
- Once the sweetener is incorporated, beat on high for 2 minutes or until fluffy.
- Use immediately, or store in an airtight container in the refrigerator for up to a week, or in the freezer for up to 3 months. Then bring to room temperature before using.

VEGAN TACO SALAD

INGREDIENTS

For the Lentil Taco Meat

- 2 cups cooked green or brown lentils
- 1 cup finely diced white onion
- 1/2 cup water
- 1 tsp each garlic powder, onion powder, chili powder and cumin
- 1/2 tsp each oregano, paprika
- salt and pepper, to taste

For the Tofu Sour Cream

- 1/2 cup soft tofu
- 1 tbsp apple cider vinegar
- 1 tbsp lemon juice

- 1 tsp garlic powder
- pinch of sea salt

For the Salad

- romaine lettuce
- diced avocado
- diced tomato
- corn
- black beans, pinto beans or refried beans

Preparation

- To make the lentil taco filling, add the diced onion and spices to a skillet with a few tablespoons of the water. Cook for 5 minutes over medium-high heat until soft and fragrant. Add the cooked lentils and the rest of the water and cook for a few more minutes until the lentils are heated through and coated in the spices. If needed, add a bit of extra water if it starts to dry out.

- To make the tofu sour cream, blend all the ingredients together until smooth.

- To assemble the salads, add a handful of romaine lettuce to a bowl then top with avocado, tomato, corn and beans. Add a couple tablespoons and about 1/2 cup of the lentil mixture to each salad.

Easy keto protein coffee

INGREDIENTS

- 6 oz espresso or brewed coffee
- 1 tbsp coconut oil or butter
- 2 tbsp heavy whipping cream
- 1 scoop of your favorite protein powder (I like to use Isopure because it's 0g carbs)

Preparation

- Mix all ingredients in large mug and combine with frother or immersion blender

- Alternatively, shake ingredients until fully combined in mason jar with lid